I FEED MY PAIN

AASHU JAIVIR

authorHOUSE®

AuthorHouse™ UK
1663 Liberty Drive
Bloomington, IN 47403 USA
www.authorhouse.co.uk
Phone: 0800.197.4150

Published by AuthorHouse 02/04/2016

ISBN: 978-1-5049-9954-0 (sc)
ISBN: 978-1-5049-9955-7 (hc)
ISBN: 978-1-5049-9962-5 (e)

Contents

Dedicated to all my students

Pain is temporary. Quitting lasts forever.
—Lance Armstrong

Preface

This book is my attempt to explain why people are not fit despite the availability of unlimited literature on exercise and diets. Why is it essential to work on your mind before your body? What are the elements that can make you dynamic and motivate you to achieve a healthier lifestyle? This book will help you gain an insight into what you might be doing wrong and what is keeping you away from your targets. It will shed light on the psychological barriers you have to surmount and show you the practical way to be fit for years to come. Using the simplest ideas to bring out the extraordinary you, this book will help you visualize and access your inner strength. You will be able to identify the negative patterns in your fitness regimen and never again fall into the trap of short-term, quick-fix regimens that give you no long-term benefits.

Balance of Thoughts

Balance is such a simple word, but it defines the core of your attitude towards life. It also determines the steps you intend to take to improve your situation in life. Someone once told me that our thoughts become actions and our actions become our lifestyles. Clearly, it is immensely important to have a balanced thought process, regardless of the result. You will understand this better by reading the chapter. Herein, the term *balance of thoughts* means consistency in your thoughts and actions over a long period of time. In the context of fitness, consistency in thoughts is affected by a person's varied experiences; boredom arises from repetitive activity and the expectations it creates. This kind of boredom is common after following the same routine day after day, year after year. This often seems to happen to people who have achieved their initial targets but who fail to carry their success forward. At the same time, your own attention, dedication, and involvement in your activity increases your expectations. If the results do not meet your set expectations, you tend to lose your enthusiasm and slip away from your path midway. This vital change in your thinking breaks the consistency in your schedule and pushes you to give up the hope of achieving your target. It is a common story with each one of us. This is what makes balance of thoughts very important for us, year after year.

Who does not wish to look good? Even you must have thought about the question at some point in time. Everyone wants to look good, and everyone enjoys admiration and appreciation. The desire for admiration is fuelled when we compare ourselves with celebrities. They make us realize the importance of having good physiques, as theirs not only help them earn a lot of appreciation from everyone but also make them stand out in the crowd.

People tend not to hold the same attitudes towards anything for the long run. The attitudes I am referring to are basically our perceptions of all the situations we face in life. You will not deny that we all are victims of our own circumstances, which often force us to change our opinions and modify our actions. Therefore, our current points of view might differ from those we will hold about the same things in a few years. Humans do not have the sort of foresight that can accurately predict the future. This makes it next to impossible to keep our thoughts consistent for a long time. Our thoughts change according to our experience. One of the most obvious examples of this tendency is our eating habits. We subtract many things from our diets and add others to them over a period of time. The story is same with our exercise regimes as well. On the first day we start our regimes, we always expect to continue with them all our lives, but a majority of us bite the dust very soon and fail to continue what we started. This causes an imbalance in our thoughts, a volatile factor in our lives.

For example, all the big stars with good physiques, such as Salman Khan and Aamir Khan, are good examples of dedication to goals. They may be on opposite poles in many aspects, but if their attitudes towards fitness are compared, they are actually very similar. The consistency in their thoughts about the well-being of their bodies is their formula for success. Yes, you might say that they are paid to look good, but doesn't a fit and healthy body make you confident and get you much-wanted attention? Even after twenty years in their profession, they are quite adamant about their fitness regimes. Think of the way they looked twenty years ago, before they decided to improve their physiques. Looking back, could you ever have predicted that they could improve so much? In their case, professional pressure also created several hindrances to continuing their regimes, but their consistent focus and strong-mindedness has made them what they are today, helping them carry themselves on par with actors who are almost half their age.

Again, I have to tell you this that there is no shortcut to success. Your fitness should be independent of what is happening in other aspects of your life. This will help you succeed if you are struggling to achieve your fitness goals and will carry you forward if you have already achieved your initial target. People can have different kinds of problems in maintaining their balance of thought; we will discuss these later in the chapter. Fitness is just like a cricket test match; even though all we are interested in is the result, we also come to realize that during those five days, there is a lot of hard work, dedication, and determination associated with the result.

Let us take the example of Indian actor Hrithik Roshan, who once commented in a press conference that before his so-called overnight stardom, he had struggled for nine long years to get the perfect body; it didn't happen overnight. What we see is the final result, but the way he is dedicated to his workout regime and still takes time to work out despite his hectic schedule is what I call *balance of thought*. When you want to achieve something and are focused, you stop trying to take shortcuts to your goal; there is just one goal of perfection you are aiming at. This powerful and channelled thought process can help you achieve the goal and carry on even after that.

Coming back to Hrithik, he must also have faced the problems of boredom, criticism from other people, and disappointment at not achieving the result many times in the beginning. Since he would have been focused on the ultimate result, he would have set many smaller targets on the way to winning his ultimate battle. It is persistence in the face of pressure that made him a star. If you have a big goal in mind, you have to be prepared to fall not once but many times. This will determine the degree of your success and give you strength to take the blows of failure in stride, giving you the courage to walk again till you achieve what you wanted to. Persistence will bring faith in yourself, while the pressure of situations or negative results will boost your strength to face all odds.

Our faith in ourselves is mostly shaken by the negative attitudes of other people or their judgmental remarks about us. No one thinks anything negative about him or herself to begin with. This seed is sown in us by others. We nurture it, and it hampers our confidence. It becomes a parasite that eats away our belief, making us judge our actions and doubt our capabilities. Criticism should be taken as manure and should make you believe that people do give attention to what you are doing. For example, it is common for people make comments like "Why are you exercising when you are not getting any results?" or maybe "Your change is not good enough". Instead of taking their comments in a negative manner, you can learn two things from them – that your efforts have already caught their eye and that your efforts may be making them insecure or jealous, because your level of effort is far better than theirs. Now the point is this: why and what does this have to do with a person's fitness?

If you are struggling to achieve some goal in fitness, there will be times when you will have trouble achieving your targets. In this scenario, persisting in your activity with a positive attitude and wholehearted effort will determine your degree of success. Always remember, the Roman Empire was not built in one day; likewise, you have got to be consistent and remain positive even if people around you behave negatively or refuse to understand your dedication. You need to fight against your own tendency to judge your actions negatively based on the criticism of others and, at the same time, to persist even when you do not see the expected result in the present. A great writer once said that it is better to fight to death than to live in despair. You too should change your attitude and the way you approach the same activity.

Sometimes the cause of your failure might be the right effort being made in the wrong direction. Here one's thought process should be balanced enough to keep one positive and heading in the right direction, rather than heading for the wrong direction with the right thought or in the right direction with the wrong thought. In either of these latter cases, the results will be negative, since both the right direction and the right thought are prerequisites to reach the ultimate goal. I have seen some women who are striving to reduce their weight or maintain themselves at a certain weight stay away from eatables so that their weight remains low. This makes sense to them, but it is completely unnecessary in my opinion. When we speak of weight, we actually refer to the total sum of four things: bone weight, muscle weight (lean body mass), water weight, and fat weight. These four are variable in nature. So two people who have the same weight cannot necessarily be considered to have a similar physiques since they could have variations among the four variables. One person might have greater muscle mass while the other could be high on fat, even though they weigh the same. Logically, we can say that a person with more muscle mass would definitely be better off than a person with greater fat content.

There is another important aspect that weight-watchers must keep in mind. I know that many people check their weight first thing in the morning, but think for a moment: can you count the number of breaths you take in one day – a most basic action that keeps us alive? Did you know that drinking even one glass of water can increase your weight on the scale by 300–400 (? How is it possible to get an accurate reading of weight? Besides, you now know that you are actually checking only one variable, and it is not practically possible to ensure that all the variables are constantly at a certain level. All that you can and should ensure is that all the variables are within certain limits.

Let us take the example of two girls of the same age (we can call them A and B) eating the same food and following the same sleeping patterns; they are of the same height, too. Now suppose they stand on the scale to check their weights. Girl A may be five to six kilograms heavier than Girl B, but Girl A measures three inches less at the waist and is slimmer than Girl B, although she is basically lighter in weight and possibly has less bone density. Now compare the two. Which one would you like to be? I don't think anyone would want to be Girl B. So why measure your fitness level by the scale? You should have other parameters by which to judge yourself. This is the situation where we are never balanced.

Coming back to Girl A, she might be committed to fitness and may take part in many activities, but at the same time, she may be sacrificing by not eating the foods she loves. Wanting to be fit does not mean that she needs to kill her desire for food or give it up completely. Sacrifice is pointless, as your periodic indulgence in what you have sacrificed is inevitable. This indulgence will make you feel guilty, and you will once again lose your balance of thought. In this case, sacrifice is a curse. I have noticed that people try to make the amount of sacrifice they make in their eating habits equal with the amount of weight loss or fitness they want to achieve. But I firmly believe that trying not to have their favourite cuisines is a negative approach and will never let them feel satisfied. The suppression of normal eating habits only succeeds in building up mental pressure, which is in itself unhealthy. Such sacrifice is not sustainable in the long run. Consistent deprivation will increase your attraction to such foods exponentially. The more you try to keep yourself away from certain types of food, the more likely it is that a day will come when you cross your limits to satisfy yourself. In fact, the most common areas of weakness for any human are food and sleep. It is hard for anyone to give up either of them. Indeed, they need only be regulated in order to achieve the desired results.

One's quest should not be to attain six-pack abs or a size-zero figure but rather to look good and be healthy over a long period of time. We must realize that an ideal figure cannot be sustained for long, and after some time, with age and hormonal changes, your body cannot respond to exercise the way it used to. Hence, what one should aim at is to be fit, flexible, and disease free after a certain age. This theorem doesn't hold true for people working towards specific targets, as is the case for those in sports or those who have some specific aim even in their later age. For example, all the film stars these days are far ahead of others in their age brackets in terms of fitness because of their consistent efforts to look good, since for them it is a professional requirement. Since these individuals have a reason to continue their same levels of activity, they do not fall into the bracket of people we are discussing here.

Now let us talk about people who have achieved their initial targets already. Such people need to choose their further actions carefully and properly so that they can maintain and improve upon what they have already achieved. The fact is that getting initial results is relatively easy, but maintaining your results over a period of time is more challenging. If you make fitness your religion and you want to be at your best, you should respect your earlier success and make efforts to sustain it with balanced thoughts. In most cases, due to lack of balance in one's thoughts, the commitment fails once the initial result is achieved. I don't think it is easy for any human being to completely avoid the problems we have already discussed or to achieve a perfect balance of thoughts. Boredom caused by repeating the same routine, as well as social and lifestyle factors, makes consistency difficult. This might result in leaving the gym, even if you have been a gym freak for some time. The reason for such a decision often lies in the absence of balance between your activities, lifestyle, and ultimate fitness goal. If you enlighten your fitness path with the necessary balance of thought, I am sure people will appreciate you even more than you expect.

To understand this balance factor, you need to think about people who have been able to achieve what you are looking for but who are perhaps ten or even more years ahead of you in the process. How do they look now? Most of them would have ended their fitness stories by losing their drive and giving up all that they had achieved. If you analyse their negative attitudes, you will find that it was the loss of a balance of thoughts that prevented them from turning their successes into long-term fitness. They may have put pressure on themselves by overdoing the exercise while restricting their diets more than necessary. Here again we can see the negative effects of sacrifice coming into play. As I mentioned earlier, you need to understand that sacrifice itself is responsible for shaking your balance and dropping you off the track.

Apart from that, what is the point of working so hard and yet ending up as a couch potato one day? No one looks the same when they are fifty as they did when they were twenty. Of course, everyone can put in the effort to look fit and healthy, and hence younger looking, like the actors do. But the point is that you must start thinking now. You need to have a positive attitude, and your goal should be crystal clear. You have the freedom to exercise the whole day, but is it necessary? Anybody and everybody can look good in a short span of time with pills, crash dieting, and working out like a freak. But rather than take these shortcuts, wouldn't you prefer to continue to enjoy the appreciation of the coming generations in your family? As we had discussed right at the beginning, it is one of the basic desires of humans to be appreciated or admired. Since we cannot separate ourselves from our desires, we need to understand our bodies, appreciate our food, and learn to exercise with the right attitude.

The outcome of imbalanced thoughts is that your body may seem fit today but your mind may be stressed. You need to constantly question yourself. Is your direction and motivation consistent enough to keep you in the bracket of fitness achievers even after a decade or more? Keeping faith in yourself will definitely set you free from other people's judgements, since you are focused on the long-term outcomes. It is practically impossible to be consistent for a very long time in spending long hours training. You need to recognize this fact and try and regulate your "high times" and "low times". The high times will be short in duration and should be marked by aggressive and very result-oriented workouts. This high time is vital because you will get maximum results in this phase. However, you should not always exercise only for the result. You should aim to improve your performance after you have evaluated and analysed your fitness every so often. You should not forget that a result is always a by-product and not the main product, in terms of weight loss or weight gain. High times should be intensive and should usually last from fifteen days to one and a half months, depending on the degree of performance improvement you are looking for. On the other hand, low times are longer in duration, usually around one and half to two months. You have the freedom to decide this duration for yourself, according to your long-term fitness plans. During this phase, you can take it easy in terms of both exercise and diet. You can avoid sacrificing your favourite cuisines and still manage to eat out by complying with your basic workout regimen, which would set you up in the right direction. You will not face bizarre setbacks or lose all that you have achieved. This cycle of high and low times will definitely keep you in action for a long time without needing to use the word *sacrifice* ever again!

Defining Horizons

After the first chapter, you understand the importance of creating a balance of thoughts, not only in attaining your target but also in maintaining consistency of effort. Now the question that arises is: how should you gain clarity of mind about your goals or what you want to achieve? What is the best way to set practical goals? How can you evaluate whether your targets are being matched by your efforts? This chapter will help you streamline your thoughts and will allow you to visualize your target with absolute precision. If you have already attained your initial targets, then this chapter will help you to continue to succeed without flatlining.

When people set targets or goals for themselves, they are often not very logical or practical. However hard they try, their efforts, more often than not, end in failure. This may have something to do with the way they set their objectives in the first place – usually by imitating somebody else's workout or aspiring to ape their dream model. If we consider such objectives in terms of motivation, these sound quite appropriate, as they provide reasons to move ahead and concrete examples of how to do so. But most people forget that any two bodies in this world are only as similar as they are different. In the first chapter, we took up the example of two girls. Taking the same example forward, we can say that they may be the same anatomically, but physiologically they will be very different from each other.

Under any given circumstances, if two people were given the same workout and diet and functioned under the same conditions, they would still not resemble each other in terms of their physical shapes. Moreover, having a dream model in mind as your target body will cause a disparity between your efforts and the perceived results. It must be apparent to you that everyone's body responds differently to the same set of exercises and the same diet. In fact, in a bid to follow someone else's regime, you lose the confidence to be the best that you can be. But you need not neglect your dream model entirely, so long as you gain the inspiration to keep moving forward.

I am sure you will now be able to analyse and think independently about your actions. Always remember that your self-assurance is the best weapon you have to counter the web of disillusioned thoughts and dissatisfaction and the lack of results.

When it comes to defining your targets, you should not forget to break down your ultimate goal into a number of smaller goals. This helps you keep track of your progress and enables you to analyse and improve your performance in the next stage. Of course, setting smaller goals cannot ensure the consistency of results based on your actions. Here you should use the services of a professional trainer. The trainer would have the experience and foresight to define your results logically and practically. Defining the target gives you a mental boost and keeps your thought process positive, thus helping you achieve your desired goal.

But the flip side to setting targets is that people often respond to them in entirely unexpected and negative manners. In other words, people have the tendency to overreact and judge their efforts too soon. They expect the reactions of their bodies to be as fast as their minds can dream. They expect change too early. If you are one of these people, then you must realize that this tendency is what keeps you so far away from your targets. In reality, this reaction to or judgement of your own efforts is quite normal. What I mean is that you tend to judge your achievements or progress more frequently than is required. You must remember that Mount Everest cannot be climbed in two days; it requires a long, sustained effort.

Also remember that your body has limitations, but you mind is free to dream or expect anything. Over time, constant cross-examination of your own efforts will make you lose confidence in your ability to reach your targets. You must use your mind to visualize the final target but also remain grounded in the reality of your body's capabilities. The lack of mind-body coordination in this respect is the reason there are more failures than successes in this field.

It is now time to scrutinize some of the main reasons why people begin to adopt vigorous activities to improve their physical well-being but end up with severely damaged self-confidence. The first and most noticeable trend I see is joining a gym just before marriage, as everyone wants to look the best on their wedding day. However, this sort of motivation is only short term. And what is the outcome? The weight and the physique post-marriage take a turn for the worse, and soon they look exactly the opposite of what they had expected themselves to look like. We can conclude that their targets were unreasonable to begin with.

The second most common reason for people to join the gym these days is as a precautionary measure, driven by their doctors' advice. Many people start having complaints regarding their weight, fitness, and general health as early as their twenties. This trend is substantiated by various medical tests, which prove that most people today are nowhere near the fitness parameters for their age. This is a clear indication of today's deteriorating lifestyle, wherein one's health quotient is below average. However, most people end up overdoing the activities, injuring themselves, and then giving up. In such a case, the activity is only used as a temporary tool to get over the distress of a situation rather than as a long-term practice with a view to perfect health. At the same time, the unhealthy lifestyle does not change, except perhaps in the short term. Thus, this exercise turns out to be a purely defensive reaction which, practically speaking, does not help the person in the long run.

Last, but not the least, some people join a gym to add credit to their social status. This particular reason is common among people of niche, higher-income groups in metropolitan societies. Here, people spend a lot just to flaunt their memberships; the most expensive trainers, gyms, and clubs get the most mileage and add the most to their status. Eventually, this attitude defeats the entire cause of fitness.

Clearly, none of these reasons should be the real aim of a workout, as an emphasis on exercise and fitness is entirely absent. There is also no foresight or desire to build a healthy future. Thus there is far less chance of achieving anything long lasting. Thinking over all the different views discussed in the earlier part of this chapter, we will realize that even though the reasons were all very different, ultimately the outcome is the same: low performance.

Most people are very resistant to change but still expect wonders from themselves. They set up targets that are too tough and impractical and forget the need to be fit in the long run. This story always ends with defeat. The solution to all the problems mentioned above is actually very basic. One needs to be truthful about the nature of the workout – that it is a practice and part of one's lifestyle rather than a means for earning social status, responding to medical constraints, or meeting any other short-term target. Moreover, you should define your targets properly, and when you achieve them, you should ensure that you continue to build on your achievements. The desire to change for the better is the key to remaining consistent. You should make sure not to limit yourself to one particular activity, which could make exercising a drag. Instead, keep switching from one activity to another, thus preventing boredom. Exercise in itself should be a source of motivation to keep one healthy and active. You can choose your activities according to your preference of discipline, alternating between going to the gym, doing aerobics, swimming, practising yoga, or participating in any other physical sports. If you wish to work on building muscle mass, losing or gaining weight, or any other specific requirement, ensure that you have a long-term perspective.

When your true reason for working out is the consideration about what people think of you, the commitment will only be short term, and results will be limited. A more rewarding experience would be to enjoy the activity itself and to compare yourself with your own best efforts. For example, when you are jogging, you should try to improve upon your own performance, in terms of time and distance. Your body will reflect the change automatically; you need not stand on the scale every day!

Motivation

Motivation is the driving force that initiates and directs your behaviour. It is the name for the basic desire that pushes one to initiate a fitness regime. An apt metaphor to explain motivation would be a car's gear system. You would agree that the first gear propels a car into motion from rest. In the same way, motivation is the basic urge that propels you into motion from a state of rest. Simply put, motivation is the mother of all actions.

In the earlier chapters, we discussed balancing thoughts and defining targets. This chapter will help you understand the need for, correct source of, and right use of motivation. Anyone chasing a particular target or dream needs a fire inside to inspire him or her to achieve an end. But you needed a spark to light that fire within you, and this particular spark is provided by motivation.

Motivation is just what you need when you are standing at a crossroads where you are unsure about the route you should take. Since it is impossible to predict the end of your route, you need motivation to propel you forward. You also need to maintain the steadiness of your action in the long run. It is very easy to see that the people who jump into the gym are all very motivated on the first day. They put in a lot of extra effort and arrange their time and other commitments to ensure that they can begin their regimes. Weren't you motivated on the first day of your activity? I am sure you were. But do we actually see many people achieving or reaching the goals they strived for? The answer is no. Keeping in mind that only a minuscule percentage succeeds, the question arises, if they all started with the same sort of motivation, what made so many of them miss their goals eventually?

The answer to this can be found in the sources of their motivation. Motivation can be either intrinsic or extrinsic. Both sources are useful if they keep you positively charged up and drive you to achieve your targets. Intrinsic, or inner, motivation arises from within, while extrinsic motivation comes from an outside medium, such as family, friends, and so on. Both can have either a positive or negative effect on your morale. Let us compare their positive and negative aspects. Our aim is to locate the right sort of motivation to enable us to move forward without abusing ourselves physically.

Whenever your inner self stirs you to participate in an activity and self-analysis shows that you are not seeking to outdo anyone else, it is a positive intrinsic motivation. But if you let your ego push you to act on impulse, it is difficult to stay focused and motivated. This is a negative intrinsic motivation. As discussed in the previous chapter, all the reasons for joining a gym for short-term results are basically extrinsic in nature. All these factors come from the outside, not from within. This is a natural human reaction to people's attitudes towards you. Even external factors may be positive or negative. The positive aspect will come from positive acknowledgments from your family, friends, and social circle. On the other hand, their criticism might compel you to take actions that may or may not be in your best interest. This is the most common negative extrinsic motivation. The negative approach always satisfies a short term urge rather than motivating a person for the long term. I hope you can now scrutinize the different approaches that inspire you to make decisions and can identify the ones that work best for you in the most positive manner. While I am not here to give you all the answers, I do hope to give you the most useful directives to help you find your best way forward.

I will now share a few examples to help you identify whether your present approach is positive or negative. Again, you must bear in mind that this is just a guideline. There are some people who make a great effort to feel self–motivated, whether it is to go to the gym or to start other physical activities. They are self-aware and know that fitness is not about achieving short-term targets but about being healthy for years. Therefore, their perception of "results" is different. But for most people, motivation is drawn from people's comments, preventive medical diagnoses, or other short-term targets, as I have mentioned in the previous chapter.

Furthermore, their effort is geared towards reaching a destination rather than developing a lifestyle. This motivation is not enough to sustain an effort, so people give up midway. In other words, their motivation is like a soda fizz in a closed bottle. When you open the bottle, the soda will last for a few seconds before becoming completely flat and lifeless.

We can discuss a few basic examples to understand the psychology responsible for giving us motivation. If I were to join a gym tomorrow because I felt lethargic and lack in energy, I would definitely notice myself feeling better due to the activity. This would lead me to slowly integrate my workout into my schedule. There would be no pressure on me to compete with anyone or achieve any sort of target. This motivation will have a good effect on my lifestyle, and the chances that I will leave the activity midway are marginal. But suppose the motivation is drawn from external sources or negative remarks about the way I look. If someone has commented on my body weight or physique or if I am perhaps very impressed with my friend's body, I would go through sleepless nights until I pushed myself to do something about it. Working on this impetus, I would join a gym. Rather than consider my body type or fitness history, I would be so focused on losing weight in as short a time as possible that I would risk injuring myself. In fact, my own motivation in this case would prove fatal! Think about it – how many cases have you come across of people who joined a gym and ended up with hurt backs or injured knees because they pushed themselves too hard without first building up sufficient stamina and proper body conditioning?

In a way, motivation is really commendable when it pushes you forward positively, but the obsession to seek fast results might prove costly. This cost might be anything from being injured to becoming demotivated and bored with the monotonous activity. In either case, you would end up having to halt your workout, thus breaking the rhythm your body had been building up gradually.

Clearly, it is unwise to exercise only for shallow results, to prove yourself right or others wrong. The sprouting of motivation is only fruitful when it is born out of the right reasons. You need to ask yourself how you will nurture your motivation. Will you be able to remain fit even after twenty years? Once you cultivate a broader idea of fitness, you will definitely boost your ability to continue to be physically active and healthy for many years to come. Rather than falling into the trap of mindless imitation, you must create your own self-motivation.

Dedication

The importance of motivation is confined to igniting your efforts to set yourself in motion. It is your dedication that plays the most vital role, as it helps you to continue with the activity you have initiated. Dedication means following a routine whether motivation level is high or low, whether or not you are busy at work or in your personal life, whatever your sleeping patterns are, and whether or not you are hungry at any given point of time. Just as motivation is the ultimate key to starting a fitness regime at any age or level of body fitness, dedication is the key to carrying this forward. This phase in your active life measures your commitment to your beliefs and your faith in yourself. Whenever we see people in their forties and fifties who look much younger than their age, it is undoubtedly the outcome of their long-term dedication to keeping fit and healthy. They have continued their activities as a pledge, even if they achieved their primary fitness targets decades ago. Clearly they understand that attaining a target is far easier than sustaining it. They come out to be the real winners, as they balance their motivation and consistency with the factors encouraging them to stop. Do you think they have the same thoughts now as they did when they started? The answer is simply no. What drives them to continue their disciplined approach even when they don't have any tangible destination to aim for? The secret is that there is no destination left for them to achieve because it is simply a practice or a lifestyle for them. The activity has been embedded in their routine now, and they are not dependant on any external targets to inspire them to move forward.

For instance, I know a man who makes it a point to go for a jog every day, even if he is out of his hometown for some days, whether for a work trip or a leisure break. The reward for his dedication to activity is that even in his mid-forties, he looks half his age, fit, and attractive. He comes across as a role model for most groups because of his dedication. He makes it a point to prioritize his workout rather than crib about lack of time. It is evident that people perpetually complain about their frequent travels or busy, late-night working hours to excuse themselves from their ongoing regimes, when in fact, it is simply a matter of priorities. When you set your priorities, fitness is usually at the bottom of your list. The outcome of this attitude is that even if you have had good results initially, they are lost due to your lack of dedication. There are many such examples all around us, but rare are the people who actually make consistent effort to maintain their levels of activity. All of us dream of being a part of the latter group rather than the former. I know a professional who works for an MNC more than fourteen hours a day. However, despite his gruelling schedule, if he misses his workout during the day, he makes all possible efforts to exercise at night. This doesn't mean that he is dependent on the gym or jogging, but he makes sure that he is engaged in some physical activity, even if it is just taking the stairs instead of the elevator at times.

Similarly, I have a few students who get up every day at five in the morning to make sufficient time for their regimes. These are certainly some of the best examples of dedication. But the individuals who have this dedication are far fewer in number than the majority of people, who have a much more laid-back perception of their exercise regimes. Since this majority can eat, sleep, and walk well, they end up overlooking the gradual changes in their posture, energy levels, and overall wellness. They get a rude awakening when a multitude of health issues arise and interrupt their normal functioning.

In this chapter, let us then study the major flaws and factors that contribute to people's falling out of the fitness rhythm. It is most important to first set priorities, as I just mentioned. For instance, any executive in a company is usually burdened with a lot of extra work that must be done within very tight timeframes. Do you think that he needs to sacrifice his personal time in order to complete the work? Do you think he has no choice but to devote all his waking hours to work? The fact is that a person usually sacrifices his or her sleep without complaint, as long as the designated work is completed on time. It is ironic that there are no complaints about the long hours of constant work even with deprived sleep and missed meals. On the other hand, no one thinks twice about sacrificing their exercise regimes. It is doubly ironic when you consider that the professional tasks have a very limited or short-lived pay-off, whereas your exercise regime will ensure that you lead a healthy and energetic life far beyond your professional career. I have seen that more than 50 per cent of professionals take a few minutes in between their working hours to smoke five to six times a day, or even more. Adding up all the time they take off, it comes to between half an hour and an hour at the very least. But if you ask them to put in even twenty to thirty minutes of exercise, they'll say they can't due to their professional and personal time constraints.

Let us look back at the examples of the two people earlier in the chapter – the person who loves to keep himself active even when he is not in his own city and the person who exercises even when he is working late at night. Consider what their states of mind would be at the end of a long day, and once again ask the question: what motivates them to exercise despite their hectic lifestyles? The answer lies in their dedication. They are definitely not trying to pursue short-term targets, as they have already achieved these long ago. You will also notice that time is never a hurdle for their pursuit of fitness. Upon quizzing them further about their dedication, they have told me time and again that even if they cannot put in their usual amount of time at the gym, they'll never fail to appear on the floor; they'll just increase the intensity of their workouts.

One thing should be clear here – we are not talking about exercising everyday, twelve months a year. A person ideally needs to put in just three to four days a week, but the important thing is to ensure that this minimum level is always met. It is my belief that such people are motivated primarily by their self-perception. Since they have a different point of view, they think and act differently, and therefore they look different. Here, *different* means above or better than average, as compared to people in general. The true factor that sets them apart is their thoughts. They are motivated to turn their thoughts into actions, leading to their overall improvement.

Suppose you sacrifice the leisure time that you usually spend with your friends to go to the company's gym. Your friends may initially be resistant to this change and may even call you mad or crazy, but this is where you need to make your choice. If you prioritize your workout, you will soon earn the appreciation of your friends and hence strike a healthy balance between fitness and your personal life. An added advantage would be that when you met your friends next, you could enjoy your food, unlike others who are always counting calories. It is a fact that when we try to make positive changes in our lives, even our friends are more than happy to give us negative feedback and lower our morale. It is basically their myopic view that makes them do so, as they recall their own unsuccessful efforts. They had clearly already lost the mental battle and were neither motivated nor dedicated enough to make an effort to succeed.

The other side of the story is the people who did achieve their targets following all the basic rules but who are now finding it extremely difficult to continue. Some of the reasons that they face problems later are very pertinent to our discussion. Like many enthusiasts, they start their regimes positively, fulfilling all the prerequisites to reach the success podium, but they eventually slide back and lose all that they had gained. For example, suppose someone follows all the required steps to reduce his or her weight – including doing the prescribed exercises and maintaining a restricted diet – for six months and ultimately achieves his or her goal. But in the end, if he or she gains it all back, that person is a very good example of a highly motivated but non-dedicated being. I do not think that such people are actually missing out on any of the elements to reach their goals. All they need to do is to prioritize their fitness and manage their time accordingly. They would certainly succeed in their endeavours and remain healthy for the long run.

Attitude

An individual's attitude is the predisposition to pursue an activity. In the context of fitness, these actions are responsible for the result of your fitness regime, whether positive or negative. We can also say that your attitude is the orientation of your behaviour that is developed after succeeding or failing at your efforts. In this sense, your attitude is your behavioural response to your workout and is therefore a basic reflection of your commitment to changing your fitness outlook and becoming healthy. This is the factor which defines your character. This chapter attempts to identify the pros and cons of achieving and not achieving targets.

Your attitude is the final perception of your motivation and dedication, with regard not only to your regime but also to how you behave publicly. The attitude is not limited to any specific reaction to a given situation, like the few we have discussed in earlier chapters. It is much deeper and broader. When discussing dedication and motivation, keeping your exercise and diet in mind, it is your attitude that guides your core actions. The reactions or responses might be positive as a result of a particular action, but the roots of the attitude embedded in you are truly responsible for wholesome change. It is not a short-term, goal-oriented process; rather, it is the measure of how you perceive yourself and how your character is perceived by others.

You must be wondering why we are even thinking about and discussing such a factor, which seems to have no connection to exercise or dieting habits of an individual. In fact, there are two reasons for this: First, the results of your exercise have a deep impact on your self-perception. Second, your attitude defines other people's interactions with you. If I were able to improve my self-image by looking the best I can, my self-confidence would get such a boost that other people would be influenced as well. On the other hand, if I were unhappy with the way I looked, or if my energy levels were low, it would make me defensive and hesitant in approaching anyone. Naturally, people would react the same way toward me. This is why it is mandatory for every one of us to succeed and feel appreciated. Of course, fitness is the best gift you can give yourself, but I don't think anyone would love to have a body which is not appreciated by others.

But there is yet another aspect of individual attitude visible in those who succeed. You must have seen people who succeeded and then began to behave in a pompous and condescending manner just because they got to their finish lines. This is a common enough phenomenon. For example, have you ever seen body builders walking on the road? They walk rather strangely and stiffly just because they are so proud of their bulging biceps. I am certainly not demeaning them, after having worked myself as a fitness expert for over a decade. I do acknowledge their hard work, but I would like to point out that being fit does not mean you need to exhibit an awkward stance and stiff behaviour. What people often do not realize is that the way they walk and talk can give out negative vibes when they are so full of their own success. Now, that is a negative attitude. It makes them conceited, and they go against all the public display etiquettes of good human beings. Obviously they were not like this from the day of their first workouts. They become indecorous only after achieving results. While they should certainly be proud of their achievements, they need not go overboard.

As I mentioned earlier in the chapter, everyone needs to be appreciated, since appreciation gives you satisfaction and a thrust to keep you going. What good would Amitabh Bachchan's or Aamir Khan's best acting performances be if they didn't have any fans left to appreciate them? Aren't they successful? But have you seen them behaving rudely in public? Since they know that their identities and success are subject to their behaviour in public, they are careful and down to earth despite their tremendous popularity. Clearly, it is not their acting and hard work alone but also their behaviour in public and their attitudes towards the adulation they receive that are important. I have already mentioned how people affect you in the chapter "Balance of Thoughts". In fact, I believe that the objective of fitness is not only to change you physically and make you socially appreciated but also to make you a good human being.

Let us also discuss our attitudes towards exercise. Does your attitude actually play a crucial role in your end results, and is it really instrumental in the continuation of your regime? To answer this, I would like to share with you the example of a very successful businessman whose attitude not only helped him achieve his target successfully but also aided him to continue. He is none other than Mr. Anil Ambani. His dedication to staying healthy was impressive even before he commenced his fitness regime, but after reaching his initial target, he transformed his life into an endless fitness routine, maintaining and improving his levels of fitness. He is full of confidence and determination. This makes him seem even more committed and self-possessed. Whenever there is a marathon in the city, he is the first one at the starting line. He doesn't need to participate for the publicity or to advertise his presence. I don't think he is any less busy than any one of us. Indeed, he is running a multimillion-dollar company. Thus, it would not be surprising if he faced a time crunch. Despite this, he takes time out for himself, which is reflected in his positive attitude. Similarly, the legendary actor Amitabh Bachchan is said to be very dedicated to maintaining a high level of fitness. It is quite a well-known fact that after finishing his shooting schedule and social commitments, he sets aside some time every day for his exercise, even after crossing the age of sixty. This is an example which directs us to be positive about our regimes.

But we do have another category of examples. There are many people who are not able to continue their success stories, as they become defensive after achieving their targets. The main reason is that they are scared of losing what they have acquired or earned. For example, I have a student who showed remarkable weight loss but who began to behave negatively towards maintaining a high protein intake and pursuing weight training. This is the outcome of a lack of knowledge of fitness and a fear of losing one's edge. Fearful of gaining weight again, she has cut down her diet to stay slim and is paranoid about gaining even a few grams on the scale. This is not what is called a positive attitude, even if you are adhering to your regime. It is certain that with such a frame of mind, you can barely survive for a few months or years as a fit person. Instead, you need to be positive and seek knowledge from the experts instead of starting or stopping anything that you feel affects your results or regime.

Once you are well educated about true fitness, you will be in a position to set rules for yourself. These rules will gradually become ingrained and will manifest as your attitude. Another very popular figure you should consider is Sachin Tendulkar, who has been playing at the international level for over two decades now. During this time, many other players have come and gone, but he has remained consistent, fit, and focused. This is all because of his attitude towards the game. All the examples that I have shared here reflect that an individual's positive attitude towards fitness will naturally affect all other spheres of his or her life. Not only will you develop a distinct and impressive personality with such a positive attitude, but you will also become a better human being. History gives us ample proof that any successful person who does not have a good attitude will soon bite the dust. You do not need to model your life completely on the people whose examples I have given here, but the idea is to put in the thought and effort and work to achieve a positive attitude and a positive outcome for life.

Guilt Factor

In the first half of this book, we discussed several important concepts, like defining your horizons, developing a balance of thoughts, and having motivation. In this chapter, we will discuss the main reason for people's inability to achieve their goals. It may come as a surprise that most people are themselves responsible for not attaining their targets. They get deflected from their path because of many factors. Fitness enthusiasts do not lose the battle when they don't achieve what they aimed for. Rather, their surrender occurs before that, when they loses their will to strive for their goals because of different situations. This creates feelings of guilt and makes it more difficult for them to remain objective about their actions. On the other hand, if you gain motivation from the difficult situations you face rather than losing your will because of them, then you will definitely witness a success story. Let us try to understand how and why different people react differently to the same situations, resulting in either success or failure.

If you think of your fitness life as a long marathon, the guilt factor acts as a speed breaker or rumble strip in your mind, preventing you from moving forward. If these strips are stronger than your will to move on, your target will always be out of reach. This explains your approach to your guilt. If your will is strong enough to overcome the guilt and handle it effectively, then you are on the right path to success. Guilt is basically the outcome of our indulgence in any activity which breaks the rhythm and pattern of our fitness regimes or diet schedules. You need to develop a great deal of mental strength to counter your guilt and move ahead to learn from your past experiences and mistakes. You must have noticed that nowadays every sports team has their own psychological therapist to help the players handle the pressure arising from the games. In the first chapter, I emphasized the human tendency to sacrifice things only to later overindulge as a result of the deprivation. Whenever we give in to this tendency, we feel guilty. Not only have we broken our rhythms, but we do not enjoy the break either because of the guilt. To move forward, we need to handle our guilt in a deliberate and confident manner.

All of us love food. As I have already mentioned, sacrifice is impossible for the majority of people. No matter how long you manage to keep away from your favourite food, one day you will end up eating it again. If you are fond of spicy or non-vegetarian food or have a sweet tooth, you could certainly sacrifice it all in a bid to be committed to your activity. But how long do you think you can realistically resist before your resolve grows weaker and weaker and you finally break? When that happens, you'll feel like you have cheated yourself and will question your self-control. This is where guilt develops, at what I call the breaking point. It is the point where you start resenting having given up something, so much so that you move from not doing anything about it to protesting by overindulging. This story is applicable not only to your diet but to your workout regime as well. Often, when you are unable to sacrifice your pleasure-seeking and lazy tendencies and end up missing your workout, you start feeling guilty. This breaking point usually manifests as a negative expression of emotions within us. Psychologically, it is very destructive for us. For example, I may break my diet, go out for a meal, and feel guilty later. I'll then spend a lot of my time complaining and worrying about my break from discipline. This makes me feel bad about myself and even negates the momentary happiness I had gotten from my meal. How many times you have done this? Frankly, these instances or events never really end in our lives, so this breaking point becomes familiar to us.

The consideration here is not what you indulged in but what your perception was. No negative reaction towards yourself is acceptable. All it does is lower your confidence. Likewise, anyone who is concentrating too much on calories, in the context of either exercises or disrupting diet patterns, will have paranoid thoughts of their own degradation. In the end, it becomes a major issue and distracts you from reaching your goals. In my view, if you think along such lines, even after being regular with your activity and committed to your diet, then your fitness efforts are pointless. Your efforts of exercising, getting up early to make time for your regime, or sacrificing your favourite delicacies while dining out with your friends should definitely be worth more than that. Remember: do not give guilt more importance than it deserves.

The mind tends to draw your attention towards worst-case scenarios, and even a small deviation from your regime can cause you tend to think negatively. I am sure you would agree that if the end result of exercising so religiously is to feel this way, then it seems rather pointless to put in the effort at all.

When you realize that you are reaching the breaking point, where guilt arises, you need to consciously take steps to counterpoise your own misdoing. In fact, we shouldn't even call it a "misdoing," since you enjoyed it while doing it. We should go to the greatest extent possible to accommodate our desires without hampering our regimes. So, you can enjoy your food without feeling guilty about it. When I take a break from my regime and eat out, I make it a point to enjoy myself. But at the same time, I prevent guilt from taking over by tailoring my diet and regime over the next few days to counter any ill effects. In this way, I can maintain the fitness of my body for years. So don't think that one doesn't need to work hard to pay for any indulgence; just prepare your mind to be strong enough to work it all off.

Remember that your efforts at fitness are not justified if you don't feel happy or can't enjoy things that you like. First and foremost, be positive about whatever you enjoy. In my entire professional career, I have seen that people either behave like fanatics, trying to run away from food to maintain their regimes, or else they cannot survive the resistance and complain constantly. The reason for these varied responses is simply perception. How do you want to perceive your regime? Sometimes, overthinking your actions and intentions makes you judgmental. I have seen that overanalysis can sometimes completely paralyse one's thoughts. In such a scenario, you just need to relax, put aside your guilt, and focus on your next step.

Correct Actions

In this chapter, we will discuss the application of everything you have learnt up to this point. In a way, all the previous chapters can be considered theorems, whereas this chapter provides the actual practice. Not only this, you will also realize the few basic problems we face in assessing a person's fitness regime. What would you say if you found out that whatever you had been practicing in terms of fitness and diet over the years was not only wrong but also self-destructive? You would be shocked and would then ask "why does everyone do it if it is incorrect?" The things requiring correction may range from wrong diet patterns to sedentary lifestyles. The latter is common in metropolitan living, while we inherit some of the dietary and genetic tendencies from our families.

Sometimes these factors are very difficult to change – for instance, we may have to eat the same food as the other members of our families at the dining table. A child sharing the same food as the rest of the family would grow up to resemble them as well. The blame for this is usually put solely on genetics or family history, but we should not ignore the fact that what we eat has a profound effect on our physique as well. By the time a person reaches adulthood, he or she is trapped in a food pattern which seems impossible to break. Most average Indians in their late thirties look the same in terms of their bodily appearance. This is because the norm is to have carbohydrate rich meals, which start showing their effects only by the thirties. In the same way that smoking and drinking are recognized as slow poisons, one's food patterns can also be seen to have a very significant negative effect on one's immunity and fitness. Furthermore, if a child was sent to study abroad at a young age, in Europe or America, it is more than likely that he or she would not resemble the rest of the family so much anymore. More than the internal factor of genetics, it is the external factor of food habits that determine how you look and how healthy your body is.

It is common knowledge now that the diseases plaguing people over thirty include high blood pressure, hypertension, and diabetes, all of which usually have some relation to dietary practices. The question then is, how can we maintain our fitness and immunity through our youths, through middle age, and right up to the time we are old? What is the factor that causes the trouble in the first place? The answer is quite simple.

The culprit is our usual practice of consuming carbohydrates late at night. Ideally you should not eat a large meal after six o'clock in the evening if you have a low metabolic rate and eight o'clock if you have a high metabolic rate. So an early dinner with very small portions of carbohydrates (carbs) would be a great way to control fat deposition in your body. Instead, you can definitely increase the portions of proteins and fibre. Think of it this way: eating carbs at night is like filling your petrol car with diesel. If human beings have been created as natural machines by God, we need to recognize what the correct fuel is for us to function in the best way possible.

We all live very similar lifestyles. Our time is divided into getting up, eating, sleeping, walking, and doing every other thing we do. This pattern is always backed up by our psychological understanding and reactions to anything we do or anything that happens to us. Just as we discussed the effects of carbohydrates, I would like to contemplate the effects of several basic lifestyle situations that can affect our health in the future. We need to understand the sources of energy used and needed by a human body. A human body draws energy from three things – the food we eat, the sun, and finally, oxygen, the most important element in keeping humans alive. All these are freely available, but we as humans never truly understand their importance.

To start with, people often wake up late in the morning. If I had to count the people I know who actually make the effort to get up early, the number would be almost negligible. I am quite sure it is less than two percent of the entire number of people I know. And yet, this is the first step you should take to start your day right. You should make an attempt to find a logical reason to move your exercise regime to the morning. Whether you read the Vedas or listen to fitness gurus, you will notice that everyone talks in different languages and ways, but all are unidirectional about regime timings. All the yoga gurus organize their sessions in the mornings, even though they know that they would have greater attendance in the evening. But the real reason why yoga is always conducted in the morning is that the oxygen levels are very high at that time of day. That is why everything is fresh in the morning, while at night everything seems so dull. Biologically, we already know the importance of oxygen. No human can survive in its absence for over a few minutes. There are almost three million chemical reactions occurring in our bodies every second, and for every single reaction, we need to have the pure form of oxygen. The only time the earth provides us with pure oxygen is in the morning. So it makes logical sense for any fitness guru to suggest that you take up exercises in the mornings. Doing so also provides a tremendous feel-good factor. This good feeling will not only start your day nicely but will also keep you high on positive energy throughout your day. Of course, exercising in the morning is always preferable, but remember, even if that cannot always happen, you must still take out time for your regime anytime you can during the day. Take advantage of your motivation and dedication to continue your regime.

One of the most frequently and widely discussed topics related to being fit is diet correction. We have also discussed it briefly in the first half of this chapter. As I have already suggested, you can blame the carbs in your dinner for your weight gain. Total fitness is about 80 per cent diet and 20 per cent exercises. Keeping yourself off carbs at night ensures that your body corrects its internal balance, helping your organs function properly, as well as improving your muscle definition. It is human psychology to blame eating out for any disruption in body weight. People often make it sound as if someone had put a gun their heads and asked them to eat unhealthy food. The first step is to acknowledge that we ourselves are responsible. Let us do a quick calculation. If you eat two good meals in a restaurant per week, that makes a total of eight restaurant meals per month. In a month, you eat about ninety meals, which means that you eat eighty-two meals at home. Even if you increase your dining out frequency further to ten or twelve times a month, how can you prove that the few meals you ate out actually made you gain weight? In fact, you eat more frequently at home, and thus it is the diet at home which should be blamed. If you make more of an effort to ensure that your meals at home are balanced with appropriate amounts of proteins and fibre, you will soon see the difference for yourself. I am sure you will be more than satisfied, since you won't have to feel guilty about eating out anymore.

On the other hand, there is one social malpractice that is common in society: accepting invitations from friends and relations and sacrificing your regime. While being social and spending time with people is perfectly fine, it is imperative to be aware of whether these get-togethers have any negative effects on your regime. These are people we are close to you and who are supposed to be your well-wishers. That is why I sometimes find it strange that these same people are often responsible for the disruption of our fitness. As I already said, eating out once in a while will not upset your system. The trouble is that with friends and relations, eating out can become a daily occurrence, especially during long-drawn events like weddings. You need to be aware of your body, make sure you eat only as much as your body wants, and give it the workout it needs. The smart action would be to take time out to perform your activity even if you don't think there is enough time. When you have to spend time with people, it may be a good idea to involve them in your workout as well, thus helping both of you! One of my students successfully follows this policy. Whenever he has to go out for a few hours in the evening with his friends, he still sets aside a little time to be at the gym. He does a quickie workout and then rejoins them later. Thus, he doesn't miss his regime and still spends time with his friends; that way everyone is happy.

I did mention the energy of sunlight, too. However, I am not suggesting that you should be out in the sun in the afternoon. As with oxygen, early morning is the best time to benefit from the sun's rays. Seeing the sunrise not only gives a soothing and cooling effect to your eyes but also relaxes your mind. You can go through any religious books and you will find the same appreciation and importance given to the sun. Can you imagine the earth without sunlight for some time? Everything in this world would become stale and dead. The sun is the source of natural positive energy given to us by God.

Once you are ready to put in the effort, the next important action is to follow instructions correctly. We need to understand the significance of professional instructions. For example, I had a client who was having problems understanding the basic instructions of working out. Some people might experience this as having difficulty directing their activity to achieve the optimum results. Unfortunately, most people are somewhat conceited and do not want to admit that they have doubts or that they need some help. As a result, they tend to continue doing the wrong actions and may even end up harming themselves.

As I mentioned earlier in the chapter, one of my clients started out well and achieved a good level of fitness. He then wanted to improve his physique further. However, he was quite reluctant to take protein supplements. He did not understand that the needs of his body had changed with his workouts. Because he neglected the increased protein requirement, his muscles did not get the fuel they needed, and his efforts did not bear fruit. In such cases, even after hiring a trainer, the required result will not be achieved unless you make use of your trainer's experience. If we think of our bodies as buildings to be constructed, proteins are the bricks that we require to make strong structures. The vitamins and minerals act as the cement. How can you make a good building unless all these elements are provided in the correct proportions?

Think of your trainer as an architect. Once someone told me that the problem with people is that they never follow professionals; they just hire them. Remember, your trainer is your guide, and he or she will minimize your efforts for better results in the long run. Therefore, trust in your trainer and make the effort to gain as much knowledge and experience from him or her that you can. You will certainly achieve your fitness goals with ease!

Myths

Our minds always play games with us by creating psychological boundaries and restricting our will to cross them. In this way, self-myths are generated, causing you to state your boundaries without ever thinking of pushing them. In this chapter, we won't be talking of the normal myths, which this book has already clarified. Rather, this chapter will attempt to point you in the direction that you normally neglect; it will be a stairway towards self-realization and will highlight the importance of being independent.

To begin with, just think of a person reading a fitness schedule on the Internet, in a newspaper, or through any other medium. We always tend to follow the instructions attached to attractive pictures, imagining that we will soon change our bodies to look like the ones in the pictures. For example, carefully observe this picture and read the instructions written alongside it.

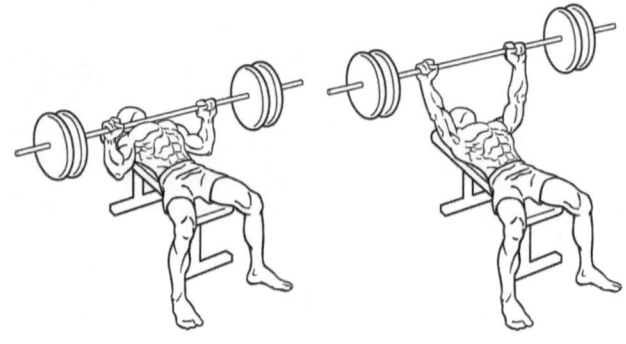

It is very easy to believe that you will achieve what is being illustrated, since no beginner actually understands the core requirements needed to reach the target. At that level, we are totally unaware of what is to be done. Think of yourself in the first class of a new subject. You would certainly need time to get acquainted with the new subject. Similarly, we rely heavily on the information available via the Internet, in articles, or through other media. For example, I have known many men who buy Arnold Schwarzenegger's *Encyclopaedia of Body Building* believing that they will be in Arnold's shoes someday soon. I find this very naive for the simple reason that his genes, the climate in which he worked out, and his diet are extremely different from their own conditions and circumstances. If you actually think of all these factors, you will realize that none of these conditions matches with those of the Indian subcontinent. His genes are strong enough to support such workouts, and the diet he followed was suited to the cold conditions he lived in, as opposed to the tropical climate of India. Along with this, he built up a very strong bone structure, which enabled him to maintain so much extra flesh. I don't mean to imply that you can't get close to what he looks like, but as mentioned in the chapter "Balance of Thoughts," no two bodies in this entire world are identical. To prove my theory, you can start your regime together with any of your friends. Have exactly the same diet and follow the same workouts for a period of time. You will find that you and your partner don't match a bit. That is why expecting yourself to become Arnold is a myth for you, even if you follow his entire schedule.

Instead, you should keep your body, your targets, your environment, and your diet patterns in mind when you have to follow an regime to which you are unaccustomed. Always remember the following pointers whenever you read an article or write-up about fitness solutions:

1. Read the fitness material, but keep a focus on locating solutions to your specific needs. Remember, many such articles will tend to have very generalized answers.
2. Read all available material on any given topic in order to widen your perspective further, rather than blindly believing the first article you come across.

I hope the importance of what you read and how you apply it to your regime has become clear. I have been featured several times on fitness shows on TV and was surprised to note the kind of questions the anchors would ask me, like, for example, the following:

- Winter is coming. What should one do to maintain one's weight?

- What is the best diet to follow to reduce weight in winter?
- If someone wants to lose ten kilograms, what should he or she be doing?

Each of these three different questions has the same, generalized answer. But how is it possible that one kind of workout could work for every individual, no matter how different people are? When you are looking for a perfect fit, you go in for custom tailoring. The ready-mades of any brand, no matter how good, still need to be fitted by your own tailor. Similarly, your exercise schedule needs to be customized to fit your specific requirements. The chapter "Correct Actions" has already touched upon the common regulations that everyone should keep in mind to achieve perfect fitness.

Another major myth that I have come across is attached to the psyches of people who drink and smoke. Having failed to control these habits, such people constantly recite the following excuses to the world:

1. I can't jog anymore (or I can't jog for very long), since I have so many cigarettes every day.
2. In the last few months, I have gained so many kilos because of drinking.

These are the most common reactions, and I hear them from almost 50 percent of people in these situations, since this is the general perception of many people. It seems to be true as well from a medical point of view. There is no doubt that both drinking and smoking affect your stamina and cause weight problems. But let's try, for an eye opener, to see how much water the above mentioned justifications actually hold.

It is not unknown that there is a world of difference in the thinking and attitude of a civilian and that of military personnel. Both the excuses mentioned above are the legacy of civilians who want to justify doing whatever they feel like doing. In these excuses, no action is taken either to eradicate the cause of the distress or to validate the truth of the reasons given. But if someone who believes these statements to be true is asked to participate in some activity, he or she hides away, citing these two reasons. Such people fail to realize that somewhere along the line, they have to pay for what they are doing to themselves. It is this defensive attitude that I address. In my experience, almost all retired military personnel drink and smoke every day, but I have never seen any of them cribbing about weight gain or reduced stamina. Then why are such problems faced by most of the civilians? The answer to this conundrum is concealed within the basic thinking in the two groups. In the armed forces, discipline is the basis of the daily routine. This helps military personnel to stay in control and balance their fitness perfectly. There are many different rules that they follow, but two of them might be like the following:

1. If their discipline includes walking every day, winter or summer, whether it's raining or not, they never miss their walk.

2. If they are trained to get up at a particular time, they will always get up at that time, every day, irrespective of what time they went to sleep.

As you can see, following just one particular discipline keeps you so motivated that you actually have the freedom to eat and drink freely, which is the one thing that everyone wishes for in this world.

Almost everybody places a lot of importance on warming up before exercising, and they make sure that even if the workout time is cut down to half, they never miss their warm ups and cool downs. This is a positive and correct way of approaching exercise. It not only flexes your muscles and makes it easy for you to work out better but also saves you from injury.

But there is still one question in my mind which needs answers: what do we mean by fitness? Let's say you can run for 10 miles or can lift 100 kilograms with your chest and even more with other body parts. People generally measure their fitness according to such parameters and consider themselves to be fit. On one level, I appreciate this, since that means they are able to perform their activities as per their expectations. But this is not a convincing or complete definition of *fitness*. I believe fitness is your body's readiness to perform in different situations or to withstand extreme conditions. I think I can sum all that up in one word: dynamic. In my opinion, you should work towards making your body fit enough to perform in drastic and rough situations. This would be the ultimate charm of your fitness. The way people usually work on their bodies makes them defensive, and this negative mindset makes it difficult to face extreme situations. Think of a situation in which you are being chased by a mob, and you have got to run for some miles to save yourself. What would you do? Would you run to save yourself or warm up first, since you would be running fast? Doesn't that sound funny to you now? This is true for when you are being chased by a mob and in many other do-or-die situations. I hope you now have a clear idea about what am I referring to. As a last, hopefully helpful allegory, think of someone being chased by a dog and running to save himself or herself!

Everyone can and should have the dynamism to be able to perform well in drastic situations. It is evident that some people run every day for many kilometres and build up their stamina, but they can't lift any weights. This is truer with women. They restrict themselves psychologically, thinking that they will gain muscle mass if they undertake weight training, which is biologically incorrect. On any given day, they might actually end up hurting their backs by picking up, say, a bag weighing 10 kilograms, or even by picking up their own babies. An example of a totally opposite kind is that of the body builders who may lift tons of weight but who would have a very difficult time if they had to run for a few miles. In both situations, the people in question think they are fit, but this is a false perception. It doesn't mean that they are wrong in performing their activities, but when your body demands effort in another aspect, you should recognize the need and work on it. Your body should be able to withstand pressure; that is what I meant by *dynamic*.

If you are exercising to be fit, then you should keep in mind the following:

1. Be dynamic. You should be able to perform any task at any time without restrictions or mind blocks.
2. Don't practice only cardio or only resistance training.
3. Don't make a schedule or set a target for yourself; take the help of a trainer.
4. Don't try to justify your weakness of will; instead, work to rectify it.

We should think of amending our thoughts and starting fresh and healthy journeys. You should make some rules for yourself. Know that these will certainly be difficult and painful to follow. The next chapter speaks about some such rules that I made for myself; they will surely help you to make yours.

Anthem

You must be wondering if we have discussed every possible aspect related to fitness in the preceding chapters so that we can get the book over with, but there is still one aspect left to be discussed. It is the one which separates the strong from the weak, the brave from the cowardly. It is as important as the adrenaline which drives you to perform beyond limits. This aspect is called *willpower*. Every human being has been gifted with willpower by God. This willpower gives us strength to fight against all odds. Even if you are motivated or dedicated to the greatest degree, your willpower will always have a major role to play in actually achieving your target. In the previous chapters, we have discussed the common weaknesses we all have, our shortcomings, and the steps to overcome them. Our basic judgments about any situation should be analytical, and each one of us should identify what is right and what is wrong. Then the choice is ours. But mostly, we end up choosing the wrong actions that lead us to dead ends simply because they seems easier and show results for the short term.

Generally, there are two categories of people in terms of fitness. In the first category are the experienced people, and in the second are the newcomers. The first kind of people will make things happen, crossing every hurdle they come across in order to keep up their regime, even while others give up. This willpower helps them to unleash the inner strength that every one of us possesses. Some of us use this gift in daily life, and that serves to separate the strong from the weak. Willpower is completely unintentional and instinctive, since it is a part of our behaviour or lifestyles. Every single day we take some actions which are part of our systems and which we need not think about at all, like getting up at the same time or maybe having dinner at a particular time. That's what I call our lifestyles. I believe that it is our thinking that makes our lifestyles. Now, these thoughts are called "self anthems". Just like every country has an anthem and every school has a motto and a morning prayer, we really need to have such defined rules in our personal and professional lives. Some of them have been naturally embedded in us since birth, and the rest are the outcome of circumstantial behavioural patterns. The latter are altered by changes in lifestyle and socio-professional experiences. In common language, we can call them *habits*. These habits are deeply ingrained in our systems, and in the case of wrong habits, they are difficult to break.

Speaking of habits, you must have realized that every one of us keeps talking about his or her habits. If anyone is asked to get up early, the most common responses are "I can't, since I slept late" or "I can't feel fresh in morning". This was just one example, and I am sure you can come up with many more if you consider it a little longer. These habits will definitely affect one's willpower to perform or achieve any result. At the same time, there are people who don't want to miss their morning walks even if the weather is not good or they don't really feel motivated about it that day. For them it is always "I have to go for my walk". Both responses can be seen to operate according to different kinds of anthems. In the first case, the anthem is being used as a defensive mechanism, while in the other case it is used in the absolute opposite way. Surely the anthem, if functioning as it does in the second case, enhances your willpower and will encourage you to continue your activity. As I mentioned earlier, this willpower would be important to making you a stronger individual who is a self-believer and who remains fit for many more years.

Even if we realize the weakness of the willpower within us or recognize that an anthem is counterproductive, we still tend to resist fresh thoughts. However, all that really means is that you need to change your anthem and improve your willpower, even though it is not easy. There are two reasons why this is not easy – first, we are weak, and second, we find it difficult to adopt change. This is common, average human behaviour. But then again, we always wish to make our identities unique among others, even though in contradiction we keep following ordinary rules.

This is mostly because of self-pampering and average outlooks and attitudes towards any action or decision making. Human behaviour is always geared to find a comfort zone and stay away from hardship, struggle, and pain. Self-pampering, an average outlook, hardship, struggle, and pain are signs of your fall into the common resistive human response. The self-pampering provides the easiest means to satisfy ourselves without struggle, hardship, or pain. But still everyone demands to be unique and better than others. For example, suppose some of us reacted to a delay in dinner. We would behave as if we might die in no time without food. Likewise, sleeping just a few hours less will always make you feel as if you don't have the energy even to stand for a few minutes.

These are all self-destructive anthems that limit your thoughts and restrict the dynamic growth within you. Change in this case lies in devising new anthems or habits with correct analysis and will power. If you start thinking about surmounting the limitations, you will become dynamic and will surely feel unique among others. Here I can help you a bit to think of your anthem. Here are some that I often use:

1. I hate myself.

We are only in dire straits because of self-pampering, as I mentioned above. To bring out the best in you and keep that going for long periods, you need a certain degree of self-hatred. This hatred means that you need to hurt yourself to the levels of saying no whenever your heart demands a yes. There is no free lunch in this world. Even if I prefer to have pizza, I can't afford to have it for every dinner just because I like it. So I might listen to my heart maybe once a month or more. But I always ask myself two questions: Have I earned it? Will I be able to balance the calories which I am taking in?

Surely it is your will power that provides you with such strength. I like to push myself till there is no energy left in me. I believe that people are average or unsuccessful in their results because they don't hate themselves enough. It is important to analyse yourself to know when you are supposed to say no. Not only will you feel the difference, but you will also surely achieve what you expect out of yourself.

2. I don't care.

Having been a trainer for over a decade, I have often come across the same excuses given by people for not attending morning exercise sessions. The basic reason they give is that they sleep late, so they couldn't possibly feel fresh and energetic in the morning. The story is no different with unwanted dinners as well. Most of us will excuse munching whatever comes through, since we wake up late and can't resist hunger. Both these examples just reflect our weakness and a lack of persistence in our commitments. Do we ever think of that when we oversleep by two hours or add an extra meal in a day? We sleep and eat our entire lives. How logical is it to give importance to missing out on one meal or some hours of sleep? We continue to nurture our weakness. Most of the time it is not our bodies which lose the will to continue but rather our brains. Our bodies are directed by our brains, so we should have the attitude of "I don't care" towards ourselves and our laziness. This approach eradicates weakness. It provides self-confidence and belief and gives us the will to carry on, even in unfavourable circumstances.

3. I love killing myself.

I have seen people questioning their trainers and blaming them for what they have not achieved in terms of fitness targets. But the majority are at fault themselves. They always see others and imitate them and yet expect themselves to be different. Moreover, a trainer can be with you for your training period only, but what you do with yourself for the rest of the day can make you or break you. Even during training, I have seen people wasting time talking in between their routines rather than concentrating. There is no merit in a long workout without intensity. They may feel satisfied that they have spent ample time on the activities, but this still leads to failure. You should train yourself for pain; then there will be no way that you could fail in your attempt. It is always a challenge to outdo yourself, but it is rewarding, as long as you secure yourself from any undue injury.

All these are examples of the sort of anthems which always instil in me the willpower to remain committed to myself and my well-being. They give me the strength to overcome my own challenges and reconsider my limitations. It is essential that we devote ourselves to new rules in order to bring about a change in our thinking and to achieve new horizons in life. After reading the entire book, you should be successfully ruling your body with your mind to achieve whatever you have dreamed of. To sum it up, you need to wake up from the sleep of laziness and low motivation and put in the effort to explore the path ahead to reach your dream goals.

Appendix 1

Case Studies

Having read the book, you now have a theoretical grasp on the steps that you should take to achieve your fitness goals. In this section, I share with you several case studies that demonstrate how those theories can actually be put into practice.

While the names of the people have been withheld to maintain privacy, the events described are completely true and based on my own observation. As you will see, you too could succeed in your goals the way these people did.

Case Study 1

The first case is of a girl who was completely undisciplined in her diet and exercise patterns. She used to exercise three to four times a week. Her exercises included aerobics or dance class followed by a short session of yoga. Despite all her efforts, she was not able to tone her thighs, which she saw as her problem area. She constantly reiterated "I can eat everything, and I don't get fat," but she also repeatedly proclaimed her negative belief that "I can exercise as much as I want, but my thighs never show any difference". Thus, she continued to exercise sporadically, not achieving any constant or appreciable results.

Analysis: After acquiring her inputs, I observed her and saw that, in fact, her lower body had more energy and was far more toned than her upper body, which was far weaker than it should be. I then focused on her diet, and noted that she was extremely fond of spicy food. However, she was also undisciplined about her eating schedule and often binged at night. Despite all this, it surprised me to see that she was not in very bad shape, as one would expect. Her primary problem was a lack of focus. She could not bring forth the required concentration to prioritize her workout and overall fitness while balancing her diet.

Action: This was quite a difficult case since the problem was not restricted to her actions alone. Instead, her entire attitude needed to change. To begin with, she was very difficult to deal with. She was resistant to a change in thinking and constantly repeated the two proclamations mentioned above. To deal with this one-track thinking, I asked her to stop sporadically doing aerobics and yoga. Instead, I put her on the treadmill to ensure a good cardio and weight training workout. Throughout this period, she was resistant and unwilling to give up on her pet beliefs.

This case illustrates that if you are following a certain pattern or regimen but not getting results, then logic dictates that you should change the pattern of how you think and act. In the case of this girl, the day she changed her fixed beliefs, she saw a tremendous change in her levels of fitness. To achieve this change, a person often needs the intervention of an expert who can clearly identify the need and guide him or her through the process of the change. On your own, you would tend to function according to your preferences rather than your actual requirements.

Result: A few days into the new regime, the girl began showing tremendous change. In fact, the results were far better than my expectations. She stopped eating junk food at night. She was regular with the workout I had recommended, putting her own ideas and preferences aside. Within a short period of two weeks, she felt the difference in her thighs. She gave up her previous negative attitude and has been steadily maintaining herself ever since.

Case Study 2

This case involves a working professional who had always been busy with his work schedule. However, he was now striving hard to take time out for his workout. He is one of the most dedicated people I have seen in my professional career. This man worked for almost fourteen hours every day in the office. He also drove himself over seventy kilometres to and from work. Despite this punishing schedule, he was very committed to maintaining his fitness. His problem was figuring out how to arrange his time in such a way that he could manage to have an effective workout that would not overtax his body.

Analysis: He was definitely very passionate about his fitness goals and prepared to put in the required effort. However, despite his strong will, he could not join a gym, since that would simply add more hours to his already packed schedule. Not only would it be an unbearable strain, but this kind of a system could not have been maintained consistently. Clearly, his problem was not confined to eating the wrong foods or having inadequate workouts. He wanted to fine-tune a workout system that would not only meet his fitness goals but could also be sustained on a daily basis.

Action: He did think of joining a gym, but could not find the time to invest in it every day. So, he came up with a fantastic idea: creating a small home gym. He asked for expert opinions and services so as to make the optimum use of his home gym. He also installed only that equipment that he required to meet his fitness target. He was very regular in his workouts at his gym, and his problem was solved.

Result: The only thing I can say about this case is that this man looks thirty years old, even though his age is touching forty. Not only is he fit, but his attitude and dedication are reflected positively in his body, too.

Case Study 3

This case is not like the last one where the inability to work out was caused by a packed work schedule. In this case, the problems were all self-imposed and lifestyle related. This girl worked as a content writer with a news agency. She used to get up at nine o'clock and then rush through her tasks in a frantic attempt to complete all her work. However, because she was always in a hurry, she was not able to do anything in a satisfactory manner. She used to work out every day for almost two hours. She focused on weight training, as she had a heavier upper body with thin legs. She was stringent about her diet, but despite all these precautions, she could not stay in good shape.

Analysis: Since the content writer had been using the same format of training for a long time, her efforts were no longer giving her the desired results. She was low on morale and had lost faith in her ability to change. Furthermore, her lifestyle had an immense impact on her morale, adding to her misery and leading her to believe she was incapable of finishing anything she started.

Action: To combat her lifestyle problem, I recommended that she start her day early. As a result, she started getting up at four thirty in the morning and jogging for more than ten kilometres every day consistently for more than three months. This was followed by a newly designed workout with a special emphasis on plyometrics. With an increased metabolism, she stopped punishing herself when it came to food and developed a more positive outlook.

Result: Her physical appearance improved substantially, and her body became quite balanced. But more importantly, she was now habituated to waking early in the morning. Consequently, she was able to do everything on time. This brought about such a profound change in her lifestyle that her work targets were also positively affected. She was no longer rushed for time every day. Moreover, she had developed a healthy attitude towards food, as she now understood how to burn it off the right way.

Case Study 4

This case is remarkable, as it follows the complete transformation of a young man from an overweight medical student into a fit, good-looking, and popular guy. He was overweight and very low in confidence, spending most of his time studying. Therefore, he didn't have much time to dedicate to his body. This made him into a very unpopular, ungainly guy who came across as a wannabe. This also made him believe that it was impossible for him to achieve his dream of participating as a model in the intercollegiate fashion show.

Analysis: Since he was very dedicated to his studies, it was clear that he had very strong will power. This made it possible for him to follow the difficult path to achieving fitness with complete dedication. His sole concern when he came to me was that he had a very short period of time to get in shape before the fashion show.

He required an exceptional workout for exceptional results, and that demanded exceptional efforts on his part.

Action: He started jogging regularly, building up his stamina and pushing his boundaries. He worked out every single day, never giving in to the thoughts of taking it easy or giving up. He was extremely determined to achieve his goal, and my job in this scenario was to make sure he did not try to take any unhealthy shortcuts. The right efforts alone can give the best results.

Result: He lost around sixteen kilograms in forty days. He achieved an unimaginable shape, and his physique had really developed well. His efforts transformed him both externally and internally, so much so that he was adjudged "Mr Fest" in the intercollegiate competition. Thus he became popular not only in his college but also in many other colleges, and he became a very well-recognized face. This was undoubtedly the result of his commitment. So focused was he about his fitness and diet that once when he ate a sandwich which was not in his diet plan, he called me up to ask how much extra jogging would be required to burn the extra calories. Hearing his queries, a lot of people would laugh at him, but later the same people appreciated and felt proud of his efforts.

There was no looking back for him after that. However, the most inspirational fact of the case was that even when he weighed over a hundred kilograms, he was jogging for over eighteen kilometres every day. When I asked him where he got so much energy despite being so heavy, he replied that he had watched a French football legend playing. That made him realize that if the man double his age could be so fit, then there was no reason for him not to achieve a better physical condition as well. This mental strength gave him the power to take himself to levels most people only dream of. However, it should be noted that throughout the process, I kept a sharp eye on his progress, ensuring that he defined the activity and prevented any injuries.

Case Study 5

In this case, I will be telling you about a mother of two. She had medical issues. But not only did she prove the doctors wrong, she also brought remarkable direction to her own life. She was diagnosed with hypothyroidism, and it was declared that she could not lose any weight. As a result, she was out of shape and looked much older than her age. In her case, any weight loss would have to be medically safe.

Analysis: Normally a person who is diagnosed with hypothyroidism would be low in confidence. In fact, most people mentally give up the battle at the outset. In this case, too, the woman was low on stamina and did not know the appropriate diet to follow to improve her situation.

Action: It is not stated anywhere that patients of hypothyroidism cannot lose weight, but they do need to be extremely careful and particular about their dietary choices. Moreover, their condition demands that they expend about 30 per cent more effort than any other normal person to achieve an optimal weight and fitness target. I respected this woman's mental toughness and dedication.

Once she made up her mind to get back in shape, she struggled for more than a year and a half, working out with complete dedication. Even though the efforts did not bring about any quick results, she continued without getting disappointed. Her stamina and fitness increased exponentially over this time, and she was able to run on the manual treadmill for 107 minutes, which was quite a record!

Result: As a result of her tireless efforts, she was able to control her thyroid. She became slim, and her dedication to working out and maintaining a balanced diet helped her become a successful aerobics instructor and personal trainer. She completely disproved all the people who believe that hypothyroidism is the end of a healthy and fit life.

Case Study 6

This case story concerns the efforts of a teenage boy who was successful in reducing his weight by about twenty-one kilograms in thirty-nine days. He was a young lad finishing his senior secondary examinations when he decided to work on his physique. He loved good food, knew nothing about working out, and was not very physically active. Moreover, his passion was to cook delicious food.

Analysis: There were no specific major issues in his case which could have complicated his weight loss efforts. He was a normal teenager who had never felt the need to actually change himself. However, when his personal circumstances called for doing so, he took on the challenge seriously.

Action: From a lazy young boy, he changed into a very active person. He started coming to the gym twice a day. To my surprise, he even started following the correct diet pattern I had suggested without cheating on it. He worked out with focus and energy and continued to push his body to reach even higher levels of fitness.

Result: As I mentioned above, he lost twenty-one kilograms in the correct way and, at the same time, improved his lifestyle. He continued to cook after that, but he stopped overindulging. The moment he realized that he should not eat any more, he would resist the urge to binge. With his new self-awareness, self-control, and discipline, he was a different person altogether – more confident, focused, motivated, and dedicated.

Case Study 7

This case is an example of dedication and commitment for more than a decade. This woman had been modelling for several years, but then she took a break. However, after more than three years, she wanted to resume modelling. To do so, she wanted a new look physically, as she had now entered her thirties. Although she still had good vital statistics, she knew that the modelling world is very competitive and thus wanted to enhance her fitness further. Whereas most models never consider returning to the fray, she was full of confidence and drive. Her fitness level was unmatched.

Analysis: She had not considered going in for weight training, as she was not looking for weight loss. Instead, her focus was on toning her body to the best possible degree. However, I saw that to achieve the best results, she needed an extreme workout using weights. Most women are sceptical about lifting heavy weights, and it took some time for her to be convinced. At a personal level, too, this was one of the toughest jobs I had undertaken, as there was hardly any room for errors of judgement on my part.

Action: She started weight training with heavy weights and put less emphasis on cardio. Her programme also had a good mix of plyometric movements.

Result: After just two months of training, she was noticeably fitter and more toned. She became an inspiration to others in the gym because of her new look. I was also very impressed by her self-discipline, as she did not touch non-vegetarian food throughout the duration of her programme. She was confident enough to go for a photo shoot, which included beach shots. She looked stunning, even more so than when she had been in her twenties.

Case Study 8

This is the story of a man in his mid-thirties who wanted a well-toned body. He regularly played football over the weekends and as a result had high endurance levels and stamina. Despite this, he was overweight and was not in good shape. The reason for this was his uncontrolled diet. He had never been to a gym before and had never worked on his muscles. Initially, he was difficult to deal with, since he thought he was already doing whatever was required.

Analysis: The man was good at what he had been doing, but he was not actually doing much to help develop his physique. He did not have much muscle mass in his upper body, even though football had toned his lower body. The real hurdle to overcome in his case was convincing him to trust in my judgement. Even though he approached me for help, he was guided by his own ideas about fitness. He also had the tendency to read up on the Internet and take tips from other people's discussions rather than focusing on his specific case and requirements.

Action: I started with his weight training, combining it with infrequent cardio sessions. I asked him to stop playing soccer for a while to increase the strength of his upper body. But my main concern was his diet, as he refused to follow the diet plan I had recommended. Even after two months of training, he had barely lost an inch on his waistline. When he questioned me about the result, I asked him to at least stop having carbohydrates at night. He continued to work out with regularity, but still there was not much change. I asked him once again to modify his diet a little by removing butter from his diet. Though he refused to do this, he did finally agree to cut down on carbs. Again, after a month, he complained that he had only lost a quarter of an inch. It was only when he became upset at the lack of results despite his constant efforts that he finally surrendered and agreed to follow my guidance.

Result: To my surprise, he started following the diet plan, and within weeks he succeeded in reducing ten inches. It seemed as if the extra fat from his body was evaporating. He started looking ten years younger and has been more active ever since. Once he achieved this new level of fitness, he started jogging regularly as well. In fact, his excellent physique and fitness made several of his friends very jealous. But I would say that was not a high price to pay for what he achieved!

***

All the cases mentioned above are stories of the real efforts made by people. I hope that you too will be motivated after reading these case studies, but remember, do not imitate them blindly. Each one of these people followed a distinctive programme based on the diagnosis of a professional trainer. They achieved their targets as a result of their determination, positive mindsets, and hard work. They struggled and in the end found better, improved versions of themselves. You too can achieve the same but only under the right guidance and by following the apt programme.

Happy working out!

Appendix 2

Calculate Your Body Mass Index

Body mass index (BMI) is a measure of body fat based on height and weight that applies to adult men and women. You can calculate BMI using the Metric Imperial BMI Formula:

$$\textbf{BMI} \ \ \textbf{kg} \ \ \textbf{m}^2 \ = \frac{\textbf{weight in kilograms}}{\textbf{height in meters}^2}$$

The metric BMI formula accepts weight measurements in kilograms and height measurements in either centimetres or metres.

$$1 \ metre = 100 \ centimetres$$
$$metres^2 = metres \times metres$$

Calculate BMI and Find Weight Status

Table 1: BMI Weight Status Categories

BMI	Weight Status
< 18.5	Underweight
18.5–24.9	Normal
25–29.9	Overweight
≥ 30	Obese

Calorie Burning Activities

Calorie burning activities are different for different people. A lot depends on your fitness level and your ability to push your body and mind. Given below is the approximate amount of calories burned by a 64 kg person doing various activities.

Activity	Calories Burnt
Walking 3.5 km/h	183
Walking 5 km/h	233
Walking 6.5 km/h	284
Jogging 8 km/h	518
Jogging 10 km/h	670
Running 12 km/h	800

Activity	Calories Burnt
Running 15 km/h	962
Running 18 km/h	1102
Bicycling 15 km/h	328
Bicycling 20 km/h	538
Swimming (25 m/min)	368
Swimming (50 m/min)	691
Aerobics, step training, 10 cm step (beginner)	406
Aerobics, slide training (basic)	420
Stair climbing	392
Stair climber machine	448
Skipping rope	798
Tennis	448
Badminton	420
Tennis (doubles)	308

Activity	Calories Burnt
Table Tennis	252
Dancing (slow)	154
Dancing (noncontact)	280
Golfing (with a cart)	196
Volleyball (leisurely)	196
Rowing (leisurely)	210
Ping Pong	252
Billiards	126
Croquet	168
Basketball (leisurely, nongame)	364
Snow skiing, downhill	364
Canoeing 6.4 km/h	378
Canoeing 4 km/h	196
Raking	210

Activity	Calories Burnt
Golfing (walking, without cart)	280
Bowling	154
Volleyball (game)	336
Soccer	546
Snow shovelling	546
Scuba diving	532
Rowing machine	504
Racquetball	574
Squash	574
Cross-country snow skiing, leisurely	434
Cross-country snow skiing, moderate	616
Cross-country snow skiing, intense	924
Backpacking with 5 kg load	504
Backpacking with 10 kg load	560

Activity	Calories Burnt
Backpacking with 14 kg load	658
Basketball (game)	616
Handball	644
Hiking, no load	434
Hiking with 5 kg load	504
Hiking with 10 kg load	560
Hiking with 14 kg load	658
Weight training (40 sec between sets)	714
Weight training (60 sec between sets)	532
Weight training (90 sec between sets)	350
Waterskiing	448
Ironing	140
Gardening, moderate	252
Shopping for groceries	168

Activity	Calories Burnt
Vacuuming	210
Washing the car	210
Window cleaning	210
Mopping	238
Housework	252
Waxing the car	280
Weeding	280
Trimming hedges	294
Aerobic dancing (low impact)	322
Mowing	378
Scrubbing the floor	392

Table 3: Healthy Height to Weight Ratios

Height Without Shoes	Healthy Weight Range
148 cm	44–55 kg
150 cm	45–56 kg
152 cm	46–58 kg
154 cm	47–59 kg
156 cm	49–61 kg
158 cm	50–62 kg
160 cm	51–64 kg
162 cm	52–66 kg
164 cm	54–67 kg
166 cm	55–69 kg
168 cm	56–71 kg
170 cm	58–72 kg
172 cm	59–74 kg
174 cm	61–76 kg
176 cm	62–77 kg
178 cm	63–79 kg
180 cm	65–81 kg

Height Without Shoes	Healthy Weight Range
182 cm	66–83 kg
184 cm	68–85 kg
186 cm	69–86 kg
188 cm	71–88 kg
190 cm	72–90 kg
192 cm	74–92 kg
194 cm	75–94 kg
196 cm	77–96 kg
198 cm	78–98 kg
200 cm	80–100 kg
202 cm	82–102 kg
204 cm	83–104 kg

Calorie Counts for Common Foods

Table 4: Calories in Drinks (Alcoholic and Non-Alcoholic)

Item name	Quantity	Calories
Tea (2 tsp cream, 2 tsp sugar)	1 cup	70
Tea (2 tsp skim milk, 2 tsp sugar)	1 cup	45
Coffee (2 tsp cream, 2 tsp sugar)	1 cup	70
Coffee (2 tsp skim milk, 2 tsp sugar)	1 cup	45
Cola Drinks	350 ml	145
Ginger Ale	350 ml	115
Beer, regular	350 ml	150
Beer, light	350 ml	100
Gin (86 proof)	43 ml	105
Gin (80 proof)	43 ml	93
Rum (86 proof)	43 ml	105
Rum (80 proof)	43 ml	97
Whisky (86 proof)	43 ml	105
Whisky (80 proof)	43 ml	97
Vodka (86 proof)	43 ml	105
Vodka (80 proof)	43 ml	97
Wines (dry)	100 ml	130
Wines (sweet)	100 ml	158
Champagne	100 ml	84
Brandy	30 ml	77

Item name	Quantity	Calories
Martini	1 cocktail glass	215
Squash	100 ml	70
Tomato Juice	250 ml	40
Orange Juice	100 ml	61
Coconut Water	100 ml	24
Apple Juice	100 ml	59
Fresh Lime (without sugar)	150 ml	5
Fresh Lime (with 2 tsp sugar)	150 ml	45
Dahi (toned milk)	150 g	90
Lassi (salty)	200 ml	90
Lassi (sweet)	200 ml	150

Table 5: Calories in Snacks/Dishes

Item name	Quantity	Calories
Kachori	1 small	200
Patty (veg)	1 piece	260
Potato Vada	60 g	170
Samosa	65 g	210
Dahi Vada	2 pieces	345
Bhelpuri	1 small plate	130
Chaat	1 plate	210
Namkeen (fried)	2 tsp	85
Mathri	50 g	200
Sandwich (with butter)	65 g	195

Item name	Quantity	Calories
Pizza (medium)	1 slice	150
Popcorn (plain)	1 cup	30
Popcorn (butter)	1 cup	55
Pancake (plain)	1 piece	74
Crackers, Monaco	4 pieces	50
Marie	2 pieces	55
Hamburger (Big Boy)	1	570
Dhokla	1 piece	60
Chicken Nuggets	6 pieces	323
Potato Chips	10 chips	115
Dosa (plain)	1 medium	125
Uthapam (plain)	1 medium	210
Upma	100 g	200
Poha	100 g	200
Curd Rice	1 plate	190
Vada	2 medium	130
Sambhar	100 g	120
Coconut Chutney	1 Tbsp	64
Pickle	1 tsp	20
Rasam	100 g	60
Coconut Rice	1 plate	368
Papad (fried)	1 piece	142
Vegetable Noodles	half a bowl	125
Vegetable Hakka Noodles	half a bowl	200

Item name	Quantity	Calories
Chicken in Hot Garlic Sauce	half a bowl	149
Sweet and Sour Vegetables	half a bowl	190
American Chop Suey	half a bowl	190
Chilli Chicken	1 bowl	285
Spring Roll (veg)	half a plate	180
Spring Roll (non-veg)	2 pieces	205
Fried Rice	half a plate	170
Chicken Fried Rice	half a plate	250
Pasta with Meat Sauce	1 serving	330
Lasagne	1 serving	433

Table 6: Calories in Soups

Item name	Quantity	Calories
Chicken Broth	1 cup	17
Chicken Noodle Soup	1 cup	75
Chicken Soup (plain)	1 cup	117
Cream of Chicken Soup	1 cup	191
Minestrone Soup	1 cup	83
Onion Soup	1 cup	27
Mushroom Soup (plain)	1 cup	129
Cream of Mushroom Soup (whole milk)	1 cup	200
Cream of Celery Soup (whole milk)	1 cup	90
Tomato Soup (plain)	1 cup	85

Item name	Quantity	Calories
Cream of Tomato Soup	1 cup	160
Vegetable Soup	1 cup	80
Lentil Soup	1 cup	126
Sweet Corn Chicken Soup	1 bowl	175

Table 7: Calories in Grains and Pulses

Item name	Quantity	Calories
Wheat Roti	30 g	105
Wheat Parantha	50 g	220
Puri	1 medium	100
Rice (boiled or steamed)	100 g	105
Rice, Pulao	150 g	180
Rice, Brown	1 serving	105
Rice (raw)	30 g	105
Khichri	100 g	215
Noodles (boiled)	1 cup	200
Macaroni (boiled)	1 cup	190
Bread Roll	1 medium	155
Bread, White	1 slice	70
Bread, Brown	1 slice	65
Cornflakes	20 g	80
Oats (quick cooked)	25 g	20
Barley (uncooked)	25 g	87

Item name	Quantity	Calories
Bengal Gram Roasted (Bhuna Chana)	30 g	110
Bengal Gram Pulses (cooked)	120 g	125
Black Gram Pulses (cooked)	120 g	125
Lentil Pulses (cooked)	1,200 g	125
Moong and Moth Sprouts	100 g	30
Urad Dal (with tarka)	150 g	154
Urad Dal (without tarka)	150 g	104
Rajmah/Chana/Lobia	150 g	153

Table 8: Calories in Miscellaneous Foods

Item name	Quantity	Calories
Sugar	5 g	20
Honey	5 ml	16
Jaggery	5 g	19
Brown Sugar	5 g	16
Jam/Jelly	20 g	55
Horlicks	5 g	20
Tortilla Chips	30 g	140
Nachos	30 g	140
Tossed Green Salad	1 serving	47
Garlic Bread with Oil	2 slices	180

Table 9: Calories in Vegetables

Item name	Quantity	Calories
Onion (sliced)	1/2 cup	23
Peas, fresh (boiled)	1/2 cup	55
Carrot, fresh (chopped)	1/2 cup	25
Cabbage (shredded)	1 cup	12
Corn (small)	1	70
Cucumber	50 g	7
Cauliflower (boiled)	1/2 cup	15
Pumpkin (cooked)	1/2 cup	25
French Green Beans (boiled)	100 g	30
Brinjal (cooked)	100 g	70
Broccoli	80 g	20
Baked Beans	1/2 cup	155
Mushroom (raw)	1/2 cup	10
Shiitake Mushroom (cooked)	1/2 cup	40

Table 10: Calories in Eggs, Meat, and Seafood

Item name	Quantity	Calories
Egg (boiled)	1	80
Egg (fried)	1	120
Egg (scrambled)	1	100
Goat Meat (lean)	100 g	118
Goat Liver	100 g	107
Beef (lean)	100 g	200

Item name	Quantity	Calories
Lamb Chops (roasted or grilled)	60 g	180
Lamb Leg (roasted)	100 g	235
Mutton Ball Curry	145 g	240
Mutton Ribs (roasted)	100 g	300
Duck (roasted)	220 g	440
Pork (lean)	100 g	114
Bacon	2 medium slices	85
Chicken, light, without skin	100 g	109
Fried Chicken	100 g	85
Chicken Breast, with skin (roasted)	100 g	160
Chicken Breast, without skin (roasted)	100 g	150
Chicken Breast, with skin (fried)	100 g	220
Chicken Breast, without skin (fried)	100 g	210
Chicken Sausage	50 g	116
Fish Cutlet	80 g	190
Fish Curry (jhol)	110 g	140
Prawns/Shrimp	100 g	200

Table 11: Calories in Fruits

Item name	Quantity	Calories
Banana	100 g of edible part	100
Mango	100 g of edible part	120

Item name	Quantity	Calories
Grapes, fresh	100 g of edible part	70
Pomegranate	100 g of edible part	80
Pear	100 g of edible part	50
Apple	100 g of edible part	60
Papaya	100 g of edible part	40
Pineapple	100 g of edible part	50
Orange	100 g of edible part	65
Strawberries	100 g of edible part	28
Coconut, fresh	35 g	150
Coconut, dried	50 g	250

Table 12: Calories in Desserts

Item name	Quantity	Calories
Jalebi	100 g	380
GulabJamun	2 pieces	280
Rice Kheer (in whole cow milk)	150 ml	300
Malpua	1 piece	200
Rasgullas	2 pieces	110
Sandesh	1 piece	60
GajjarHalwa in Khoya	1 katori	260
Fruit Salad	1/2 cup	98
Brownie	60 g	230
Chocolate Cake with Icing	1 piece	233
Chocolate Chip Cookie	1 piece	120
Ice Cream	70 g	140

Protein Content of Grains

Grain Type	Grams of Protein (% Recommended Dietary Allowance)
Soya Bean Seeds (White)	43.2 (77.1 %)
Masur (Lentil)	25.1 (44.8 %)
Moong (Green Gram) Dal	24.5 (43.8 %)
Chavli (Cow Peas)	24.1 (43.0 %)
Moong (Green Gram), whole	24.0 (42.9 %)
Udad (Black Gram) Dal	24.0 (42.9 %)
Matki (Moth Beans)	23.6 (42.1 %)
Rajma (French Beans), dry	22.9 (40.9 %)
Chana (Bengal Gram), roasted	22.5 (40.2 %)
Arhar, Tuar (Red Gram) Dal	22.3 (39.8 %)
Kulthi (Horse Gram)	22.0 (39.3 %)
Chana (Bengal Gram) Dal	20.8 (37.1 %)
Peas, dry	19.7 (35.2 %)
Chana (Bengal Gram)	17.1 (30.5 %)
Genhoo (Wheat)	11.8 (21.1 %)
Bajra (Pearl Millet)	11.6 (20.7 %)
Maka (Maize)	11.1 (19.8 %)
Jowar	10.4 (18.6 %)
Rice, hand pounded	7.5 (13.4 %)
Kurmura (Puffed Rice)	7.5 (13.4 %)

Ragi (Finger Millet)	7.3 (13.0 %)
Mutter (Peas), tender	7.2 (12.9 %)
Rice(Milled)	6.8 (12.1 %)
Poha (Rice Flakes)	6.6 (11.8 %)

About the Author

Aashu Kumar Jaivir has been transforming lifestyles of clients for over sixteen years. Apart from providing personal training and diet counselling, he encourages his clients to make healthy choices and ingrain them in their lifestyles. His education and experience in the fitness industry have given him a broad overview of different aspects of training. A firm believer in the philosophy that mind rules body, his approach is to aim for achieving a "fit body," and this makes him different from other trainers. He has also been featured in prominent fitness shows in India, as well as in lifestyle magazines. His knowledge and skills are evident in the lectures he has delivered at various fitness summits. He positions himself as a lifestyle guru and has worked with business owners, corporations, non-profit organizations, and educational organizations to promote the cause of fitness and educate people to understand its real meaning. An icon of the industry, his holistic approach to health incorporates proper nutrition and exercise practices as well as the maintenance of a healthy work/life balance.

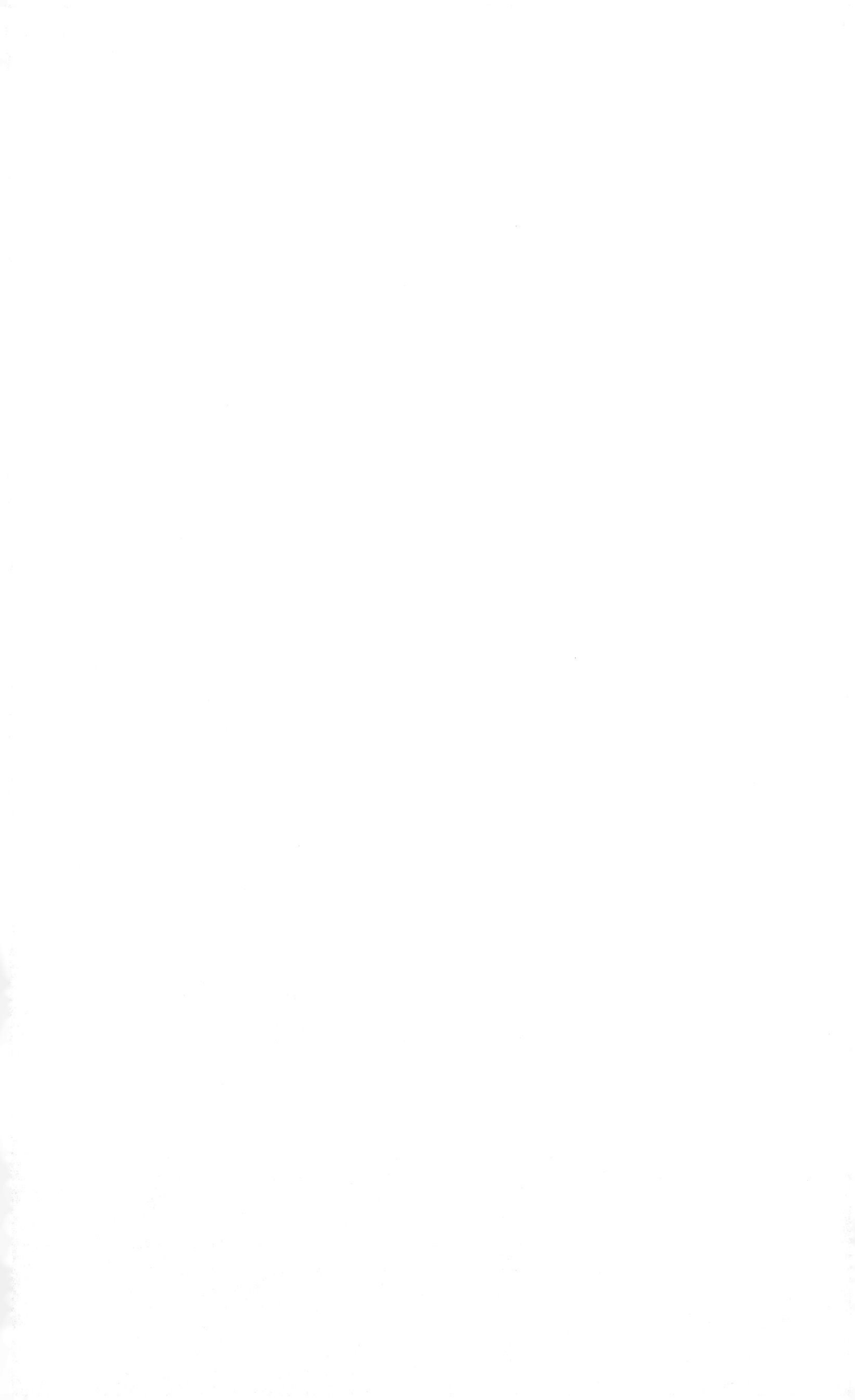